Into the Fog

Navigating My Mother's Journey through Dementia

୧୫

a memoir and a guide

by
Patty Brennan

*Into the Fog: Navigating My Mother's Journey through
Dementia* is available for purchase from Lifespan
Doulas [LifespanDoulas.com]. A 40% wholesale
discount is available for orders of six or more copies
of the book.

ISBN 979-8-9919732-1-2

To Mom,
with love and gratitude

to Mike, Peter, Joan, and John,
for sharing the journey

and to all family caregivers—
may you be graced with patience and humor

Table of Contents

Preface

I began writing this memoir on the eleventh anniversary of my mother's death in the hope that others may benefit from my stories, reflections, and lessons learned. I am grateful to have had four siblings to share the experience. Caring for Mom brought us closer. My mom had a special relationship with each of her children. You always knew she appreciated you and was in your corner.

Early on in my family's journey with Mom through the last several years of her life, it occurred to me on more than one occasion that I might benefit from reading a book about dementia or even joining a support group of some sort. Professionally, as a doula, doula trainer, and business coach, I specialize in helping folks *not* have to learn everything the hard way, through trial and error. In the face of my mother's dementia, it seemed only natural that I would take a similarly proactive approach and seek guidance for a path so many others have traveled, giving myself the benefit of their hard-won wisdom. But I did not. I suppose the prospect struck me as just another 'to do' imposed on my already stretched time, balancing work and family responsibilities in addition to caregiving. I was in the trenches, driving one hour each way at least once per week to take Mom grocery shopping and to various doctor appointments. A visit consumed the better portion of a day and a good deal of emotional energy. I fumbled my way through, trusting my instincts, sharing impressions with siblings, adapting, and learning together as we went along.

This approach worked okay, for the most part. And yet there were instances of regret—the 'if only I knew this before' moments. No doubt it would have helped to become more informed on the subject that would become a central theme in my life for several years to come. So here it is, that little guide that might have fallen into my hands but did not. While each family's journey will hold unique challenges, I trust that I have a few stories and reflections to share that might help ease your path.

Patty Brennan
May 31, 2024

The Players—A Division of Labor

I am blessed to be a member of a high-functioning and reasonable family. We (mostly) all get along well, and high drama is not our style. There was never a question that a given family member did not have Mom's best interests at heart or that one of us was not holding up our end. Nor was there any dispute or grumbling about Mom's estate, our inheritance. Everyone, without question, accepted my parents' intentions that any assets remaining upon their death would be distributed evenly among us.

Likewise, no one ever questioned my sister Joan's authority as the designated medical decision-maker. My mother's choice of Joan, who is a nurse, was intentional. In fact, Joan was chosen to be her medical proxy over my dad, when he was still alive. My father, who died more than 15 years before Mom, had designated Dorothy as his legal advocate. He made it clear that if he could no longer be expected to recover and return to work (his bottom line for quality of life), he did not want to be kept alive via machines. Dorothy, on the other hand, left a

3

different set of instructions in the event she should become incapacitated, and these can be summed up as follows: "Don't be too quick to pull the plug." While Joan was always open to input from all of us regarding any medical decisions, she assumed her authority to fulfill Mom's wishes as she thought best.

We did not always agree about this and by "we," I mean Joan and me. But I did respect my mother's choice. And so, at one point, when Mom was not yet under hospice care and consequently hauled off to the E.R. via company policy in her Assisted Living facility, she ended up receiving I.V. fluids before Joan was notified. The E.R. doctor strongly recommended antibiotics for a urinary tract infection and Joan, managing all this long distance, reluctantly consented to the treatment hoping to facilitate a quick discharge from the hospital. My position at the time was "hell no" as I wanted mom under hospice care. The result was that her condition improved and she went on to live another year and a half before qualifying for hospice a couple of months prior to her death. That last year or so was rough, as her dementia progressed relentlessly, and I had occasion to regret my sister's decision. But I have never questioned that Joan was, in fact, faithfully carrying out her assigned duty according to my mother's wishes.

There was a reason Mom chose Joan and not me.

This experience leads me to want to clarify *my* wishes at the end of life, should I have dementia, which can be summarized as 'Let me go.' Hopefully, if my wishes are honored, there will be no respirators, CPR, dialysis, forced feeding, and so on. Furthermore, I have expressly spelled out in a Living Will (and in conversation with my family) that, in the presence of a dementia diagnosis, any acute illness should be viewed as an opportunity to let nature take its course. (See Appendix C and our Resources for more information on advance care planning as well as considerations specific to folks with a dementia diagnosis.)

Each sibling contributed to Mom's care as their circumstances allowed. Mike, living in Houston with limited resources, was not able to visit in person very often, but maintained a strong emotional connection with Mom. When phone calls became too much for her to manage, Mike sent her postcards, which she enjoyed. John took over management of all her investments and finances from Washington D.C., as well as visiting when he could. And Joan managed Mom's health care, interfacing with medical providers from her home in Florida and during her bi-monthly visits over long weekends

for at least the last couple of years of Mom's life.
Peter and I held down the fort on the homefront
with lots of help, companionship, and moral
support from Peter's wife Chris. We were a well-
oiled cooperative of caregivers, with laughter
and a little dark humor easing our way.

Who She Was

How can I tell you about my mother? Certainly, she was so much more than those last few years of her life might lead a stranger to believe—that vacant shell of a being that she had become, who looked at me with suspicion and annoyance at times, no longer recognizing me as Patty, her dearly loved daughter.

My mother was a beauty, and her name was Dorothy. When I was a little girl in the 1950s, I used to love to watch her get ready for her Saturday night dates with my dad. And I mean every Saturday night. She would sit in her bra and slip at her dressing table and carefully apply her makeup. Next came the stockings, heels, and jewelry. And last, but by no means least, the dress. It was my job to zip her up. The effect was dazzling. I adored her.

My close friends growing up recall my parents' home as being "formal." A family of seven, we lived in a meticulously appointed four-bedroom colonial house in Dearborn, Michigan. Early on, my mother began to collect antiques. Her various collectibles were displayed throughout the house. One of my other jobs, besides zipping her up on Saturday nights, and

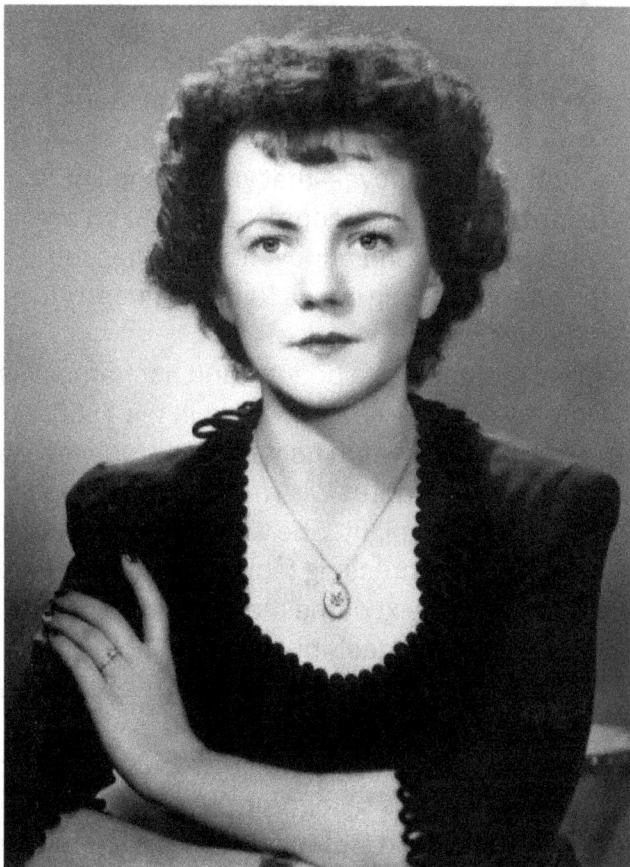

Dorothy Marie Sweeney in 1943, age 27
Newly engaged.

much less to my liking, was to dust these displays. On birthdays, we didn't simply have cake with candles. Silver candelabra flanked the cake, which was presented on a raised glass cake dish, a "happy birthday" music box magically wound and hidden within, ready to sing with the first slice of cake.

There are many more things I could tell you about my mother—how she taught us to stick up for ourselves, her love of travel, and her pride in her children. Dorothy took a vow to never say the words, "Go watch TV" to her children and she kept it. She was quite healthy (except for her poor brain at the end). She was well ahead of her time when it came to healthy eating, and she walked a mile per day through most of her eighties. She never guilt-tripped her children about not visiting or calling more often, nor did she attempt to coerce us into longer visits when we did show up. She simply was happy to see us and took delight in whatever time we had together.

But this book is not intended to be the story of my mother's life. Rather, it is about the end of her life. When did my mom's decline begin? There was a fall when she was 88 years old while climbing a step ladder to change a light bulb in her apartment. After the fall, her hip and back hurt, and she became crooked with one hip higher than the other, made especially noticeable by the uneven line of her skirt hem (she always wore skirts). She was never the same after that. Her daily walks up and down the Westborn strip mall became a thing of the past. Just one activity among many of what was to become an ever-expanding list over the next eight years.

Around this time, as she was beginning to struggle, my sister Joan embarked upon a gentle campaign to get her to leave her second-floor apartment in favor of a tiered living facility for the elderly. No more stairs, basement laundry, or carports and icy parking lots. At first, Mom resisted this move. However, she was persuaded to "just look" at a few places, no commitment to change required. In the end, Mom succumbed to Joan's argument that at this moment, *she* was in control and could choose for herself where she wanted to live rather than waiting for a crisis to occur, in which case, *we* would be making decisions on her behalf. Shortly thereafter, we moved her into the Independent Living wing of Oakwood Commons with the understanding that, should she ever become disabled, Assisted Living and, ultimately, the dreaded "Alzheimer's Unit" would be available. My mom would live out her final years in this place, one way or another.

INTO THE FOG

At first, Dorothy was reluctant to engage in the more social aspects of living at Oakwood Commons, even to the point of being irritated by the Welcoming Committee members' efforts. She valued her privacy, set her boundaries, and preferred to take it all at her own pace. From the beginning, she took her dinners in the communal dining room and gradually made new friends. She also enjoyed playing bridge.

The Early Signs

It began with her speech, searching for the right word and occasionally using the wrong one. At this stage, she could fake it, compensate, and keep her dignity intact. The problem progressed, slowly but steadily, to encompass an ever-growing percentage of lost words and cognitive connections. 'Word salad' pretty much sums it up. I can't imagine how her bridge buddies handled it (one hopes with utmost kindness and compassion). Then again, one never knows which connections are still being made. Perhaps she could still pull it off for a while at the bridge table. I began to balance her checkbook each month and marveled that her meticulous addition and subtraction skills were intact. These remained so for some time, though she was challenged to accurately track all the transactions. So, who knows? Eventually, I became aware that she no longer played bridge, but I never heard the story of how that unfolded.

While dementia is a progression, a one-way street with a certain outcome, there is a lot of bouncing around within the parameters of this diagnosis. It seems that sometimes, a certain welcome lucidity briefly returns, only to be lost again. The short-term memory goes first. Some of my mom's long-term memories, such as the home she grew up in, the church she got married in, and the old neighborhood remained intact close to the end of her life.

My brother Peter and sister-in-law Chris had gotten into the habit of taking Mom out for breakfast on Sunday mornings. Our family had traditionally gone to the Dearborn Inn on Sundays and, for a while, Peter continued this tradition. Then, one day I became aware they had switched location to the Big Boy. Peter explained he did it for the pictures on the menu whereby Mom could just point and say, "I want that" (so smart!). Justine, our server, was an important part of the Big Boy Sunday morning ritual. She remembered just what Mom wanted (same thing every week), facilitated seating at the familiar booth, stashed the walker, joked, and kept us plied with coffee, generating a sense of fondness all around. This ritual continued for several years, until close to the end of Mom's life.

After breakfast, we would load back in the car and phase two of the Big Boy ritual would begin. To extend our time together, Peter would take the 'scenic ride' home. Rather than heading directly back to Oakwood Commons on Michigan Avenue, we would tour through the old neighborhood nearby. Dorothy would often brighten up as she recognized familiar places from the past. Stopping in front of our family home on Winona, she would say, "Mine?" On one occasion, as we drove past the home of some old friends of my parents, she said, "Oh, that was so sad when that baby died." Shockingly, it was a full, comprehensible sentence, as clear as a bell—a strong memory from the past. Peter remembered the story, which I had never heard, of the drowning death of the family's six-year-old son. We continued the ride, winding our way down Cherry Hill, driving through Greenfield Village, past the horse corral, and finally home.

Dorothy enjoyed these outings. She loved going for a ride and watching the cars zooming past the window on Michigan Ave. She thought they were going *very* fast and would ask, "Did you see that?" Birds also fascinated her. Towards the end, I began to realize that her world had gotten downright tiny wherein the definition of a panoramic view had become sitting at the far end of the hallway. Being taken out afforded much more stimulation, which she clearly enjoyed.

There came a time when Dorothy could no longer manage the interface between the television and her DVD player. There was a favorite British TV series on DVD that she enjoyed watching, but she could not do the series of steps required to turn on the devices, adjust the settings, and navigate the DVD menu options. I spent an hour one afternoon drawing a map for her, with pictures and precise step-by-step instructions (1. Turn on TV; 2. Turn on DVD player; and so on). No go. (This was early on when she was still in the independent living area.) I realize now that my instructions map was a complete *non sequitur.* No doubt she was unable to even understand the connection between my instructions and, well, anything.

One day, I went to visit Mom. As I came into her apartment, she exclaimed with exasperation and relief, "Patty! I've been calling you and calling you." She was holding the remote control to the television in her hand. Poor Mom. I could only imagine her confusion and frustration that things didn't work the way they were supposed to. How long had she been trying to reach me via the remote control? I have no idea.

Eventually, the confusion extended to discoveries such as finding a used Depends hanging from the clasps of a skirt hanger and placed on the bedroom doorknob, a box of aluminum foil in the refrigerator, and so on. It was sad to think of her days consisting of wandering around, wondering where to put things, and who knows how many other frustrations.

The Goodbye Call

One morning, sometime before we moved her to Assisted Living, I received a call from Mom. She was lucid and focused and had something important to say. There was a sense of urgency about her. She told me that she wasn't always going to be here, that she could feel it (death approaching?), but it was okay. She wanted me to know that she loved me and wasn't afraid, that I should not feel bad, or worry about her. She said, "It's not now, but soon." Hanging up, the realization that my mother had just called me to say goodbye while she still could, shook me. I immediately called Joan and, sure enough, Joan had received the same call. And, as we checked in with Mike, Peter, and John, it was the same. She had called each of us sequentially to say goodbye. She lived a few more years after that.

Crisis Fuels Change

When is it time to make a change?

We can see the handwriting on the wall. We know that the time is coming when Mom should not be driving a car. Or when living on one's own is no longer a reasonable choice. Or when a primary caregiver absolutely needs relief from the physical burden of caregiving, an uninterrupted night's sleep, or respite from the relentless sacrifice of their time and energy. Sometimes, these decisions are made for us and the decision is clearcut and immediate. But often, it seems, contemplating the right time for what seems to be an unwelcome change is grey and murky territory. It is hard to wrap our minds around the fact that we have arrived at that point *now*.

Many adaptations have likely been made as we age, such as downsizing to a smaller one-story condominium or first-floor apartment. Most older drivers in my acquaintance begin to self-limit their excursions. Night driving is often the first to go. Highway driving is next. In the end, folks are just driving themselves to church, the grocery store, the bank, and other familiar places within a few miles of home. The near-complete loss of one's freedom, privacy, and autonomy, however, is another thing altogether. We put off making the call that now is indeed the time for a change for a host of reasons, including:

- Limited financial resources
- Pride
- A sense of duty
- Guilt
- Keeping a promise
- Fear of having strangers in your home with attendant loss of privacy
- Overwhelmed by the hassle of dealing with the logistics involved in a needed change
- Not knowing what to do, not knowing how to find help.

I remember a friend who was the mother of a severely disabled child. He was non-verbal, in a wheelchair, and needed a respirator to breathe. She was devoted to his care and did most of it herself. My friend was a small woman and, as her son grew into his teens, the transfers from wheelchair to bed, or wheelchair to bath, and so on, were becoming increasingly difficult for her. Then, one day, she broke her leg, slipping on a patch of ice in the driveway. During her recovery, many friends took turns helping in the home and caring for her, her son, and family. And it was through this experience that she learned to accept more help and, especially, to identify new sources of help to care for her son. Her accident spurred a necessary shift in the household and in her expectations for herself. Once they got through this admittedly rough transition, her family's quality of life improved.

Another friend's elderly sister was placed in a nursing home because she could not return to her home after a hospitalization. This was during covid when strict restrictions on visitors were in place. My friend was able to visit her sister through a window as she was housed on the ground floor of the facility. One day, my friend arrived at the window for a visit in time to witness an aide help her sister transfer from her wheelchair to the bed. When her sister did not willingly lie back on the bed once transferred, the aide pushed her down forcibly. My friend was appalled by this rough, unkind treatment of her sister and began to search for a better placement. She found a private home that had been converted into an Assisted Living type of arrangement—just a handful of residents lovingly attended by a woman who had her own apartment on one floor of the house and a more relaxed approach to covid protocols that didn't involve denying contact between family members at the end of a loved one's life.

I have witnessed a similar pattern for any number of family caregivers. If we are witnessing from the outside looking in, the unsustainability of an existing pattern of functioning and coping is obvious. We can observe the stress that the caregiver is under and the struggle of the sick, aging, or otherwise compromised family member. We see that it cannot go on and worry what might happen next. Meanwhile, the people on the inside of the situation are simply carrying on as best they can.

It seems that we are ready to face these changes when we must, when it is more painful not to change. While my own inclination is to be more proactive, I'm not convinced it is a terrible idea to allow an unsustainable situation to deteriorate until everyone can be fully onboard with the idea that the time for a change has indeed come. While solving one problem, forcing the change is likely to cause a great deal of emotional upheaval. It's a hard tradeoff. As part of the decision-making process, I do think we should ask ourselves whether inaction constitutes neglect or abuse. Is the situation dangerous for our loved one? Does she/he pose a danger to others?

Driving

For the first couple of years at Oakwood Commons, Mom was still driving. This activity had gradually become increasingly self-limited to daytime outings and nearby stores. No more downtown Detroit excursions or highway driving of any kind, but scary, nevertheless. We were constantly grappling with how/when to 'take the keys away' but that hadn't happened yet. I suppose it's just very painful to take someone's independence away, to tell them they are "too old." And, apparently, when it's *you* who has reached this point, denial is your best friend.

Peter and Joan reported several attempts and unpleasant conversations designed to get Mom to surrender her keys. She was adamantly opposed to this idea and resisted all efforts. Joan reported that Mom became sad and hurt at the conclusion of one conversation, but Peter realized (hoped?) seeds were being planted, that it was a process. The timing was such that I was in the market for a car, my husband and I having recently hit a patch of black ice that resulted in our car being totaled. Rather than argue that Mom should not be driving, a logic began to develop that Patty sure could make better use of Mom's car. By the time she finally relented and signed the title of her car over to me, Mom was behaving as though the whole thing was her idea all along. Peter reflected, once again, on the life lesson that nobody likes being told what to do. (See Resources for a *Guide for Aging Drivers and Their Families.*)

Assisted Living

One spring day, when Mom was still living independently, Peter and I realized we had both booked vacations out of town for the same week. It wasn't ideal, but we thought (hoped?) Mom would be okay in our absence. It so happened that my father-in-law experienced a health crisis just before my husband Jerry and I left for our vacation in Michigan's Upper Peninsula. Throughout our first few days away, Jerry was constantly on the verge of packing up and heading back down state, based on sibling reports. On the phone, my mom didn't sound so great either. She kept saying she just didn't feel well but she didn't know why. Finally, we decided to abandon our vacation rental and head home early.

I found Mom in her 80+ degree apartment, lethargic but happy to see me. We had been having variable spring weather, not at all unusual for Michigan, with chilly nights and mornings, and then warming up during the day. During our vacation week, a most unseasonal heat wave occurred, and Mom forgot that she could control the temperature in her apartment. She had become dehydrated from the hot temperatures and lack of air conditioning. The dehydration made her too lethargic and confused to make the trip downstairs to the dining room for meals, so she wasn't eating. This made her weaker still. She was well into a downward spiral when I found her there in this pitiful state.

It was becoming clear that Mom was no longer functioning capably in her apartment, and we began to discuss moving her to Assisted Living. It came down to the realization that it would be neglectful to leave her to fend for herself in her apartment. She needed to be taken care of. At this point in time, she was still able to participate in the decision and she agreed to move.

Key Point

When a person with dementia becomes dehydrated or sick with even a minor ailment, their dementia symptoms become markedly more pronounced.

The Move

By the time we were moving Dorothy to the Assisted Living wing at Oakwood Commons, we had already downsized our parents three times previously—from the four-bedroom colonial where we all grew up, to a three-bedroom townhouse while my dad was still alive, to a two-bedroom apartment after Dad died, to a smaller two-bedroom apartment at Oakwood Commons. I never expected it to take ten days of nonstop work for us to get her settled into Assisted Living. We did the move ourselves with our sixty-something bodies, using dollies, along with sporadic help from a couple of grandsons. An auction house in Detroit was engaged to sell furnishings and collectibles that did not make the cut.

In her new home, Mom would have no need for cooking, no stove, no microwave. A few cupboards, a sink, a small counter, and a half refrigerator constituted the 'kitchen' area. Her space consisted of a small living room, bedroom, and bath. A major downsizing was in order. We planned the move after extensive measurements had been taken with the idea of keeping as much of her stuff as was reasonable to make her new lodgings feel comfortable, familiar, and easy to navigate.

Mom was not able to conceptualize any of what we were doing. She really could not participate in the decisions, but she was still cognitively at the point where she expected to have a say, and we felt it was important to protect her dignity in this regard. Thus, the move itself became a complex psychological and physical challenge of supporting her emotionally and getting the work done in a reasonable amount of time. We endeavored to make as much of this process as possible invisible to her on the theory that 'out of sight, out of mind' and her poor memory would result in her not really missing belongings that didn't make the cut. We might have even engaged her attention at times with 'decisions' that were a foregone conclusion but nevertheless created the impression of choice and agency. Chris, unable herself to help with the physical packing and moving, took on the task of keeping Mom company and distracting her as much as possible—an invaluable contribution!

As Mom's dementia advanced, the strategy of making decisions on her behalf while protecting her from witnessing the details of us taking complete control over her life worked well.

For example, Mom owned several oriental rugs. One rug filled the already-carpeted living room, anchored in place by shelving, a loveseat, and a few other items. The rug was constantly bunching up in spots, creating a tripping hazard, and Peter and I would regularly flatten it out when we visited. Next, the rug became a receptacle for spilled bottles of Ensure as Mom would repeatedly sit on her walker, perched in front of the window overlooking a small courtyard, and fall asleep with an open bottle in her hands. After a while, the rug became terribly stained, and the apartment began to smell bad. I decided the rug had to go (we called it our 'hit list'). This task was going to require a team approach. As I recall, Joan made an extra-long hair appointment for Mom at the in-house beauty salon on one of her trips up from Florida. Joan wheeled her down and kept her occupied while the Peter/Patty team went to work in the apartment, moving knickknacks (forever plaguing me) and furniture so that we could roll up the rug. We hauled the rug out of there and put the room back just as it was. After returning from her hair appointment, Mom never inquired after the missing rug. She simply forgot about it. This would become our template for making changes going forward.

The periods leading up to a necessary change in circumstances seem to be the most tumultuous. Once we are on the other side of the decision, there is a sense of relief for a while. Whether we are faced with an aging parent who really should not be behind the wheel of a car, managing their own finances, functioning as a caregiver for another, or living independently, the decision to make such major changes will necessarily be preceded by a struggle. Sometimes, I think, we just need to let the deteriorating situation play out for a bit as we are reluctantly brought to acknowledgment of the new reality and need for action. Otherwise, how would we know that *now* is the time to make a change, especially one that no one is happy about?

Hindsight always tells the story. We can step back and map the overall arch of events and the trajectory of the decline. It becomes quite clear if we waited too long to take the keys away, hire help or respite care for a primary caregiver, sell the family home, and so on. I've come to make peace with the idea that the uncertainty and stress leading up to these decisions is okay, necessary even. We don't need to feel guilty and beat ourselves up about it. It is how the motivation to make hard changes manifests. We simply need to do our best in the moment with the information and resources we have available and accept that there is no perfect path forward.

The solutions will be different for each family and, no doubt, many factors will play into the available options, not least of which is available finances. Luckily, for my family, funds were available to pay for Assisted Living in a decent facility. My mother was 96 years-old when she died. Had she lived another four years, my brother projected we would run out of her money.

The looming specter of the 'Dementia Unit' or 'Alzheimer's Wing'

One aspect of my mother's experience in Assisted Living that created unnecessary stress for me was an overriding fear of the Dementia Unit. I remember my mom, years earlier, telling me about the pitiful condition of a friend who had been thus consigned for several years prior to her death. Having never visited a Dementia Unit, I had no clear vision of what it entailed, so my imagination conjured up an image of a fate to be avoided at all possible costs.

As my mom's capacities and ability to cooperate with caregivers continued to diminish, I worried that the Assisted Living staff would mandate a change of location for her, which I dreaded. So, it seems that, for a time, we carried on as though we were in a potentially adversarial situation in which others might force an unwanted change if Mom became too difficult, or we became too demanding of Assisted Living staff members. I was even reluctant to ask the staff questions about her care and status at times, fearing that my questions might put us on an unwanted path. In hindsight, I wish I had put this issue to rest sooner. As it turns out, I had created a straw man.

We came to learn that the philosophy of elder care had evolved and that the current trend was to keep folks with dementia in their Assisted Living apartments whenever possible. As the person's disease advances, the level of care can be increased without the need for a physical move. There are a few exceptions which make a transfer to a Dementia Unit necessary. These are:

- The person wanders, meaning they repeatedly walk into the apartments of other residents or go outside on their own.
- They become violent or verbally abusive towards others and disruptive of normal routines in the facility.
- They become completely incontinent and uncooperative with caregivers (though the incontinence itself isn't a deal-breaker and might be managed by increasing the level of care provided).

When Mom was first placed in Assisted Living, she required a basic level of care. She was continent, able to dress and feed herself, and capable of doing her own laundry. Staff took over administration of her medications and all meals were provided. She was being checked on regularly. Over the next four years, it became clear that we needed to increase her level of care when a deterioration in her condition raised new concerns. At one point, she seemed near death on hospice care, only to bounce back, be discharged from hospice, and no longer require the enhanced level of staff support. I learned that these types of reversals are not unusual for dementia patients. For families, it can feel very unpredictable and hard to navigate because it's all over the map. There is a 'What's next?' type of exasperation that sets in, accompanied by a feeling of helplessness and sadness.

It's Not Rational

She's still in there.

My mom had a strength and stubbornness in her and these personality qualities persisted to the end. Always reluctant to have her privacy be invaded or be herded into group activities at Oakwood Commons, she told me one day (in her way) "I sit here; I don't go over there." "There" was just around the corner where a chair exercise class was underway for the residents. "Here" was her perch at the end of the hall, by the dining room, where she liked to take her walker and sit, for hours on end, waiting for the next meal. I might have reasonably tried to encourage her to participate in the activity, but on some level, I recognized she was maintaining her sense of choice and personal identity, and I remember thinking, "good for you Mom, you sit right here if that's what you want to do."

She had lost a great deal, but she could still express her preferences, and this remained a consistent feature. Let her enjoy the few choices left to her.

It makes sense in her reality.

After the move to Assisted Living, Mom became very unhappy for a time. Who wouldn't be, with strangers letting themselves into your apartment whenever they wanted, telling you when to eat (earlier than you wanted to!), administering your medicines ("I can DO it!"), offering unwanted help, a third of your belongings gone. Freedom, privacy, capacity— all things of the past, but the reasons for these changes are unclear. She can't understand what is happening.

As she became increasingly confused, a type of paranoia set in, and she would often complain that something had been stolen from her apartment. Of course, the more likely scenario was that the item in question had not made the cut during the necessary downsizing involved in the move or perhaps she simply forgot where she put it. Nevertheless, her sense of violation was strong, and she was often outraged.

When she complained, my inner dialogue went something like this: *"How terrible—my mother thinks I have put her in a place where people are allowed to steal from her. Of course, I would never do that."* And then I would say, "No, Mom, that's not true. No one is coming into your apartment and taking things" and proceed to argue with her about it. I was horrified to think she believed we had abandoned her to abuse, and I set out to convince her otherwise. The argument continued for a while, escalating the frustration for both of us, as my response only served to further enrage her. She dug in her heels with the bitter accusation "you always take *their* side." More and more, it felt like our roles had been reversed. She had become the stubborn child and I the ever-so-reasonable adult. In this new reality, I had become the enemy.

On my drive home, I called my sister in tears to relate this latest sad tale. Joan helped me understand that Mom was no longer capable of a conscious thought process such as the one I was projecting onto her ("my mother *thinks* ...").

"Patty, it's not rational."

We talked about relating to her only on an emotional level. Her emotions were intact. And she feels what she feels for reasons that make sense in her reality. We must learn to suspend all expectations of rationality in our dealings with her. Accordingly, the next time she made a complaint of thievery (and in place of making it be about me), I got upset *with* her, matching her tone, and exclaiming passionately, "That's terrible! I'm so sorry that happened to you. It's just not right!" Feeling validated, she exclaimed "that's right!" and the whole blessedly short episode ended in happy camaraderie. We were on the same page. It never occurred to her that I was somehow to blame for this or had any power whatsoever over it. She just wanted someone on her side. Logic? Just another thing of the past.

Several months later, a variation on the stolen/missing items theme emerged. One day I found her in her chair all worked up about something. She kept pointing to the entrance area of her apartment. I gathered she was angry about another intrusion. Now it seems that people are coming into her apartment and leaving things there that don't belong to her! Can you believe the audacity? Specifically, a little shelf display on the wall next to the door that held two little ceramic dogs (purchased as a gift for her by my 15-year-old self while on a class trip to Niagara Falls, imagining that these chachkas somehow qualified as 'antiques') was causing her agitation. I tried distraction but she continued to perseverate on the shelf. I decided on a new tactic and said, "Mom, would you like me to take down that shelf and get rid of it for you?" Bingo! She thought that was a downright amazing idea, so I got up and easily pulled the shelf and dogs off the wall, nails and all, and made it disappear. After my exertions, we sat on her couch together while she happily admired the empty wall like I was some kind of miracle worker, saying "That looks so nice." This certainly beats arguing.

On another trip, she began to complain about the many coats in her closet. She owned about fifteen coats of various lengths and designs, suitable for every kind of weather. The theme was the same. Could I believe that people just walked into her apartment when she wasn't there and put all these random coats in *her* closet!? Peter and Joan had each been treated to a similar tirade—an ongoing stressor in her reality. But I had figured out the solution to this one. "Mom, would you like me to get rid of the coats that aren't yours and just take them out of here?" A resounding "YES!!!" was the answer. I began to take the coats out of the closet one by one, holding them up for her inspection and asking, "Is this yours? Is this yours?" One after another, the coats were rejected, a couple of them eliciting a (well-deserved) disdainful sneer. I disappeared them all into my car, to be donated. A few were deemed to be hers and allowed to stay in the closet. This made her happy.

Embracing the idea that the person with dementia is behaving in a way that is consistent with their emotions and inner reality, and that effective communication involves seeing things from their perspective and responding accordingly was a game-changer. Over the years, I have had occasion to share this lesson learned with a couple of similarly challenged friends and it helped them in dealing with their loved ones as well.

The Present Moment

I have been a midwife, a doula, a childbirth educator, and a doula trainer. Doulas are professionals who provide non-clinical support to families in transition including expectant parents, birthing women and their partners, new parents, and folks at the end of life. If there is one central, conscious, take-away message I have learned from being a doula, it is that my client's story is not my story. *It is not about me.* Now, my mother's decline was teaching me the same lesson.

Birthing and dying are times of profound change. When we are witnessing or providing support to others through these peak life experiences, our own past traumas or unconscious fears can be easily triggered and projected onto their experience. This tendency, of course, diminishes the effectiveness of our support efforts. I think we need to learn to sort out our own fears (What if this happens to me? What if one day I no longer know my own children's names and become as helpless as a three-year-old?) and acknowledge them for what they are. The horror that I am somehow looking at my own future (after all, my mom and I are alike in many ways), makes me want to push it far away. "Just shoot me" as my brother John is fond of saying. And then I remember, again, wait a minute, this is not about me. I can be as impatient as I choose, but it will not make the end come sooner any more than I can have power over the timing of a birth by wishing the baby to *be here already* for the laboring mother I am attending. It is *her* process. Her life, her birthing, living, dying, her way. It is my belief that everything happens for a reason. I cannot explain why it is taking so long nor guess when it will be over. It's just not about me. The timeline has major ramifications for me and my day-to-day life, but it is not mine. I am called to witness and help as best I can.

This realization frees me. Let her own it. I don't have to take that on. In this moment, I am free to choose my responses, and I have gratitude for my own capacity. And a deeper well of patience for her. Perhaps there is a hidden gift here I have yet to discover. It will be what it will be. Living in horror of what will come next, dreading how the process might unfold, fearing what might happen, witnessing an endless stream of painful losses and asking the ever-present "how much longer?" makes for a tough ride, one wherein we are helpless victims of the process rather than helpers.

INTO THE FOG

When a mom is laboring to birth her baby, I do not jump into her circle of pain, exclaiming "poor you." I stand apart, by her side. When she becomes afraid, I say "just get through this one." I help anchor her in the present moment. This is how we get there, one contraction, one moment at a time. I think to myself, "I've got this."

In hindsight, I look back fondly on a lovely spring day a year before her death when I put Dorothy in a wheelchair and pushed her around the flowering grounds of Oakwood Commons. I brought a 'picnic' for us—a refreshing cold drink, some chocolate, and fresh raspberries. We found a bench to rest and enjoy our treats and Mom watched the birds. She couldn't talk much anymore, at least not in a manner that made much sense, though I could usually get the gist of it. But she did still know me as someone who loved her, and she seemed quite happy. Who knew that a year later, when she no longer trusted me to take her out, that this day would become a precious memory?

Relationships, Communication, and Decline—Family Emails

My brother Peter has a wonderful, playful youthfulness about him and a great sense of humor. When stuck for a way to pass the time with Mom, Peter got into the habit of asking her about 'the picture.' He would make her sit next to him on the couch, take the framed picture in hand, and ask, for the umpteenth time, "So Mom, who are these people?" And then Dorothy would tell the story she had crafted together about the children in the picture, my first three grandchildren, James, Juliet, and baby Jack. James and Juliet were thought to be my children (not true). Juliet was a boy (not true). Jack used to live in my basement, but he isn't there anymore (true), and Juliet (he) is trying to control the baby (true!). This picture of my three little darlings provided hours of entertainment.

Email from Joan on 1/24/11:

> *She told me all about the picture of the three babies. I could tell who she was*

talking about. She did know about Jack living with Patty but also knew that "they" were getting their own house. It was all fairly coherent, even the fact that she didn't really know who these people were. She also confirmed that she had gone out with Peter when I asked her. "Oh yes, and his wife." It has been a long time since she used the right noun referring to Chris. She said she had a great time but made it clear that Peter was supposed to call her and remind her from now on. She referred to me by name while we were talking. Right away she asked me when I was coming back for a visit. But then she drifted off for a while, almost as if she was talking to Patty about me, saying that she knew there were a lot of sick people in the hospital and Joan just cannot leave them but she said she would come back for a visit. I never talk to Mom about being a nurse, so she still had that. Then she would come back to more clearly talking to me. Very strange. In and out. The main thing was that overall, she seemed happy. Several times she volunteered that everything was fine with her, that she felt good. That's good enough for me. I'll come home early in March.

41

Email from John on 2/21/11:

It was good to be home and to see Peter, Patty, and what's left of Mom. She has no clue who I am and not much of one about who Peter is (which my presence made worse) but was struck by our resemblance to each other. She could not understand why I would want to go see Patty but suggested that I play a joke on her by posing as Peter. I tried this out, but Patty caught me right away. Jerry was not fooled either. Nevertheless, Mom seemed in good spirits and enjoyed the visit. It helped that Peter came over on Saturday to introduce me. I took her to the Dearborn Inn for dinner on Saturday and got into a little trouble when I was not only presumptuous enough to order dinner for her but informed her that she liked their house salad, and that French onion soup was an old favorite of hers. This prompted her to say, rather indignantly, "You don't know me!" But it did not prevent her from scarfing down the soup and salad. I will come back sometime this summer.

Email from Peter on 3/7/11:

Joan's weekend visit was wonderful for mother. Joan, as we know, has the loving touch. Mother's difficulties bring out the best in Joan, which in turn benefits Mother. After our Sunday breakfast at Big Boy (Joan was there for the start but then had to head to the airport), Mother, Chris and I ended up back at her apartment. And, just when you think that Mother is gone and will not return, bam! She's back! She told us two stories. Both had the same basic point—how very happy she is that she and Dad (whom she unhesitatingly referred to as her husband) showed such independence at crucial times in their lives.

Story #1: After Pearl Harbor and Dad's re-induction into the army, they decide that they will not get married before he goes overseas, but rather wait, and if he returns alive, then marry. I do not remember ever hearing her state this so clearly. I thought they probably thought about getting married and probably discussed it but then decided not to marry because it was (perhaps) premature, a decision they later corrected with the engagement. But no. Apparently, they agreed before he left that they would marry if he lived. She told us this with great pride, not because he lived and they married, but because, in her view, it was the right decision. She clearly said that they saw too many people getting married so that they would have a baby in case the man died. Mother (and Dad's) view was the stupidity of planning for a fatherless child and they both just were not going to do it.

Story #2: *After John (whom she named) went east to school, she wanted to travel. She told us how happy she was to get the chance, how independent it made her feel. She reiterated the story about how Dad was all for it, not just because he was happy working, but because he too was independent minded and did not require (like too many men) the need to appear to have direct and immediate control over a spouse. She said that if her husband had objected (even, in her view, for foolish reasons), she would not have done it. The happiness, as she described it yesterday, of being independent enough to travel the world knowing that her husband supported her unconditionally, is a* *happiness that is like a Godsend. On the downside, she asked me if I ever knew her husband ... but that's a story for another day.*

Email from Patty on 6/22/11:

I saw Mom on Saturday. I brought her two packs of Ensure, some Depends, flowers, and a seasonal shelf display. She knew me and called me by name. Was very happy with the supplies/gifts and remembered the swing and the little bears, which she enjoyed arranging on the shelf. But from there, I must say it's getting increasingly pitiful. We now find a bra hanging from a refrigerator magnet; she had gone down to a 10:30 hair appointment at 8:30 and was told to come back at 10:30; when they came to get her at 10:30 she refused to go, arguing that she was supposed to go on Saturday. She had removed all the little animals from one shelf in her apartment and hidden them in her dresser drawer, claiming there were originally thirteen but someone stole one and now there are just twelve ("It's like being in hell living here"), BUT there was one left sitting up there on the shelf and when I asked about it, she said it wasn't hers and that "they" just put it there. It's just a perpetual state of confusion.

Email from Joan on 7/7/11:

As for Mom, she certainly is deteriorating. Her walking and eating and dressing are all about the same. Her speech is worse, and she only barely knew me at times. For example, when I first got there, she was just sitting down in her chair which was good because I dreaded having to awaken her. She is always disoriented when awakened in my experience. Here is how it went: When she saw me, she got a real big smile on her face and was very animated.

"I recognize you!"
"Hi Mom" (as I sat down next to her)
"What is your name?"
"I'm Joan, Mom. I'm your daughter."
"What do you do?"
"I'm a nurse."
"For how long?"
"34 years" (I find it hard to believe that myself.)
"Oh you don't look like it. I'm almost ninety."

That day she never seemed to click that I was her daughter. She didn't want to go out to lunch, I think because she was not comfortable with me. But each of the next four days, she always greeted me with either "honey" or "sweetheart" and seemed comfortable with me. However, one day she remembered that I was a nurse and asked me what kind of a nurse. I told her that I worked with patients who had cuts. She said "Joan, my daughter, does that too." Then she proceeded to express her wish that Joan would come back for a visit because she said she would. That was tough. I don't nearly mind so much that she forgets me as thinking that she misses me.

Email from Mike on 10/5/11:

Yes, Mom is still there but trapped in her brain with no way out. She knows something is wrong but doesn't know what. You can't ask her any questions. She has to initiate any 'discussion' which she sometimes does. Peter pointed at her bracelet and up from the depths comes Mildred Gridley [an old friend]. Still, she enjoys her meals, likes looking at the finches, and likes watching the trees and sunshine. I called her a couple of weeks ago. She didn't know who I was, did not comprehend the words "Mike," "son," "Houston," or "Texas." She got scared and sad. I wonder if it's worthwhile to even try calling her anymore. Peter says she does enjoy getting my postcards, so I will keep sending those although I've just about exhausted my supply.

Email from Patty on 10/12/11:

Mom continues to enjoy watching the birds. She makes up stories about what they are doing. When I went on Tuesday, someone had given her a newspaper. There's a man who sits at her table now. She introduced him to me as "the man" and he responded by saying "hello woman," which I thought showed a sense of humor. Anyway, if I could follow (which was EXTREMELY difficult), I think she was telling me that he gave her the newspaper. She seemed to think that the various Tigers players, prominently featured, were him (wearing a variety of hats for reasons that made sense to her). And the schoolgirls, who were part of another story, were the girls who follow him around. But honestly, I don't know *what she was talking about. Nevertheless, the paper was clearly providing some entertainment value, and she was making up stories about how the pictures were interrelated. Sometimes, I seem able to move away from how sad and horrendous this is, remove myself emotionally, and then find myself being curious about the process of what she is experiencing. Anyway, she still knows me and calls me Patty and is always happy to see me. But she introduces me to everyone as her sister.*

Email from Joan on 2/26/12:

Mom went into great detail about a box John gave her from Chicago that somehow people had stolen part of and left it smaller. It used to be twice as big. I don't think that is possible, but maybe that is just me.

Email from Joan on 5/6/12:

I was in Michigan last weekend. Mom is pretty muddled. She didn't really respond to me very much when I showed up on Friday. She was sitting by herself near the dining room, 45 minutes before it opened for lunch. I don't know how long she had been there. The only thing she wanted to do was to sit right where she was. She insisted that she had to wait THERE. I could not get her to roll down to some chairs so that I could sit with her, let alone get her to go out to lunch with me. After lunch (I waited in her apartment) she warmed up to me, smiled a lot, called me "honey," and said she would like to go out to lunch the next day. When I came the next day, she spontaneously called me Joan several times. She was happy to go out to lunch and we had a nice time in her very limited sort of way. The two days just couldn't have been more different. Her 'conversation' is very disjointed, often it is not English. There are times when she is comprehensible, but it is often a struggle (at least for me). It doesn't seem to bother her much.

Email from Patty on 1/27/13:

My last two visits with Mom have been disasters, both times driving an hour each way only to be (pretty much) dismissed and not able to breach the gulf of incomprehension. She is increasingly lost in a fog of confusion, and the babbling is getting harder and harder to decipher. On Wednesday, she kept insisting that she "had to go" and kept walking down to the dining room two hours before dinner. They would repeatedly tell her it wasn't time yet and we would return to the apartment. After two minutes, she would insist it was time to go again, very adamant, and I wasn't able to distract her from this, even with a back rub. On the third trip down, I left.

Email from Patty on 1/30/13:

Peter has the right idea ... a precise routine every week ... she responds well to this. Says she "will go anywhere with the man" and is very cooperative and always tells us to "come back soon" when we leave. I have recently taken to meeting Peter and Chris and Mom (often with Jerry as well) on some Sundays because it is so much less painful than the alternative for me. The only downside is that it doesn't really take much heat off Peter and Chris, so I continue to try and go in and check on her in the middle of the week occasionally or when they are out of town.

The Knee Socks

Since Dorothy always wore skirts, and pantyhose had become too difficult to manage, bare legs in the winter started to pose a challenge. Joan and I settled on knee socks as the solution. Mom had never worn knee socks in our experience so we had no idea how receptive she would be to the concept. On her next trip to Michigan, Joan went out and bought six pairs of knee socks. Five pairs were in muted or dark colors—blue, brown, grey, black, olive. The set was completed with the most garish pair of socks I have ever seen. We are talking red, purple, yellow, and orange with complex designs and *lime green* accents. They looked like something a ten-year-old girl *might* consider wearing (no offense to the fashion judgment of ten-year-old girls intended). Joan presented the sock array to Mom and asked for her opinion. One by one, Dorothy set aside all the muted, normal colors. These were accepted as fine. The garish pair were left by their lonesome as rejects, accompanied by a look of utter disgust. "Not these!" The Illusion of Choice—my brilliant sister! It reminded me of the parenting tip regarding how to handle an uncooperative toddler. "Tommy, would you like to climb into your car seat by yourself OR do you want mommy to put you in your car seat?" (Note that not getting in the car seat is not one of Tommy's options.) After Joan's clever introduction, I never heard a complaint about the knee socks. She simply began to wear them.

The Saga of the Clothes

At first, when Mom moved to Assisted Living, she was still able to do her own laundry using the shared facilities down the hall. Eventually, we had to increase the level of care and services provided to include doing her laundry, bathing her, and dressing her. The deterioration that took place leading to this decision was painful to witness. My mom was fastidious and had always taken pride in her appearance, wearing skirts and nylons, makeup and jewelry, every day for as long as I can remember. To come upon her in the dining room at Oakwood Commons dressed in an inside-out skirt, bare legs, slippers, no bra, no shirt, and an oversize V-neck sweater vest was especially disturbing and pathetic. In speaking with staff, we learned that she had worn this same 'outfit' three days running, resisting staff efforts to get her to change or put a sweater over the too-revealing vest. After this episode, I began to add select items in her closet to the 'hit list.' That sweater vest needed to go!

Peter injected some much-needed humor in the family email updates that were sent regularly, noting that on one trip to the Big Boy,

> She has abandoned any fashion concern in cold weather (e.g. mink coat with gym shoes).

In another email, I reported,

> The latest for the hit list is the multi-colored, horizontal striped knit pullover with a scoop neck. When I saw her on Wednesday, she was tugging at the neckline constantly and there were little threads hanging all over, coming unraveled. If you have a chance to grab it and toss it in the trash on your way out, feel free!

A few days later, Peter's response:

> Said sweater, having been indicted, was today duly tried and convicted of total unmanageability. Mom could not even get it on (it's a pullover) and was 'wearing' it draped over her shoulder in the dining room this morning. We took it off, replacing it with a cardigan. It has been sentenced to a spell, rolled in a ball on

*her top shelf. Final execution/destruction
may take place as soon as Joan's visit.
—PJM, Prosecutor*

Email from Patty on 2/21/13:

*I spoke with the supervisor today about
Mom's clothes. I was trying to sort out:*

- *Where are all the sweaters and a
  few other missing items? (She did
  not know about the sweaters but
  does not think Mom is giving them
  away and believes the aides would
  notice if they were finding clothes
  in the trash. So, it remains a
  mystery.)*
- *Who decides what gets washed
  and what doesn't? (Unsatisfactory
  response here.)*
- *Does anyone read washing
  instructions on the clothes?
  (Suggests we buy easy-to-wash
  stuff, no dry cleaning.)*
- *To what extent are they helping her
  with dressing? (As much as she
  will let them.)*

*I came away with the feeling that they
do what they can but don't get serious
about intervening unless it involves*

safety. We've all seen how angry and stubborn she can get. I guess this is just the deal. I think I am going to keep looking for some new clothes for her that are suitable. Unfortunately, I fear that my call may have prompted Oakwood to review her level of care.

Email from Joan on 1/26/13:

I made an appointment for Mom to get a permanent and haircut next Saturday at 1:30. Denise, the hairdresser was very apologetic about Mom's hair but said she just couldn't get Mom to cooperate. She said she goes and gets her, but Mom gets very hostile and will only go about every two weeks. Patty has been treated to this hostility. I told Denise that I would stay with Mom and try to take the heat off her. I told Denise that I want to get rid of the comb-up from the back and sides because Mom just cannot maintain it and ends up looking like Einstein or Bozo. All we can do is try. Tell Chris hope is on the horizon.

Email from Patty on 2/6/13:

There is really nothing that can improve Mom's situation. It will get worse and worse until something takes her out. An infection around her teeth due to poor hygiene there? Or a urinary tract infection? If she stays healthy, then my understanding is that eventually one loses the ability to swallow and then death follows. She is absolutely getting worse. My last three trips down have been horrible. No communication whatsoever, not even an emotional connection. Anger, hostility, confusion. My god, it's just awful to see her this way. Peter is honestly like some kind of angel with his natural, youthful humor and loving presence, but I know it wears on him as well. She continues to respond well to him, and I think it is due to the regularity and ritual nature of how he proceeds.

While Joan kept her compliant at the hairdresser's, Peter and I spent an hour and a half cleaning out her closets and some stuff in her bathroom that shouldn't be there. The idea is to reduce her clothing choices to the simplest options, getting rid of stuff that is not appropriate, stained/frayed, complicated to wear or wash, etc. We hauled out two bags of clothes to recycle and three bags of trash.

We are probably getting close to having to increase her level of care at Oakwood. The challenge is to get her to cooperate with caregivers. Though they do shower her, despite resistance. This enrages her so much that she punishes them by refusing to go to lunch afterwards. By dinner, she has forgotten. The nurse supervisor mentioned that if it gets any worse, they may have to give her some Ativan to get her cooperation with showering.

However, despite all this terrible decline, on Sunday, she seemed better and knew me again. Was very happy to see me and affectionate towards me. Terry and Sarah and the kids and Kara and Jack also joined us, so it was a big crowd. Mom seemed very entertained by all the babies, and they were sweet to her and liked petting her mink coat. When I told her I would come back, she pointedly asked "WHEN?" So, my worst fears—that she had permanently sunk into a quicksand of babbling and anger and that I had become like a staff person to her—

were alleviated. I guess it comes and goes.

Email from Joan on 2/20/13:

I think we should all take a deep breath and think about what we want for Mom. I'm sure that the drug mentioned is Ativan. Quite a powerful tranquilizer—a controlled substance. (How are they going to get her to take it?) My initial reaction was hell no. On the other hand, maybe it would be a kindness if it would make everything less traumatic for her. I do think we need to keep her clean, which is just a basic dignity issue. If she gets mad and skips a lunch, so what? This is terrible. I would be interested in everyone's opinion. It is only going to keep getting harder. Thanks Patty and Chris for your continued efforts regarding the clothes, also a basic dignity issue.

Email from Patty on 2/20/13:

Just to be clear, I was not pushing for a higher level of care. I don't understand how clothes that we just sorted out and reduced to a select few can completely disappear. I wanted to ask/alert her to the fact that perhaps they were being given or thrown away. BTW, I mentioned that I assumed she would be calling you before ever resorting to giving meds. This was not an actual pending decision, more of a warning, "if it gets worse ..."

I do not have any thoughts about medicating her, but I can only imagine the fuss she makes and how nasty she must be when they are forcing her to be bathed. My impression is that Oakwood will not allow her to be overly combative, disruptive, wandering, or unclean. If she starts heading in that direction, then things will have to change. Maybe that's when drugs enter the picture? I'm not opposed to it if necessary. But she was cheerful on Sunday, delighted even to be going out, so drugs will (I imagine) even out the anger, but we probably would lose these few remnants of enjoyment as well.

Around this time, I began to create a list of requirements for any replacement clothing:

- ✓ Dark or multi-colored tops, serving the dual purpose of disguising the lack of a bra while hiding stains due to spills

- ✓ Easy on and easy off (no buttons or zippers); elastic waistbands for the skirts and simple slip-on tops preferred
- ✓ Straightforward wash and dry, with no special care required such as dry cleaning, hand washing, or air drying.

In anticipation of Mother's Day, I went shopping for some clothes for Mom. I remember contemplating a cute, petite blouse and thinking she would like it. It had a slight puff in the sleeves, buttons down the front, and a bow tie at the neck. I stood admiring it, thinking how much it suited her and was consistent with her taste in clothes, all the while completely disregarding my list of requirements. In my mind, I was shopping for the old Dorothy, not my mother of today. I moved on, declining to purchase the blouse.

Email from Patty on 3/25/13:

> *Every time I have seen her since the big clothes clean out and increasing her level of care (they are clearly dressing her now), she has looked nice and clean and well cared for. It's these transitional phases, and leading up to them, that are particularly difficult. Her hair has been better as well. Yesterday, they had a cute*

little scarf on her and one of the new skirts I bought.

Feeding at the End of Life

M y sister the nurse had witnessed many elderly patients in her care over the years being kept alive via forced feeding, whether this was via tube feeding or by hand, shoving food into an uncooperative person's mouth. Joan was adamant from day one that we would not be doing that. 'Concerns' about Dorothy's weight were repeatedly voiced by the doctor at Oakwood Commons who urged us to supplement her three daily meals with bottles of Ensure. As Mom liked Ensure, we followed this recommendation and made it available to her.

Email from Joan on 9/28/11:

> *I took her to the clinic at Oakwood to see Dr. X because there was a question about her medications. I was able to once again impress on him that I only want "comfort care." I made it clear that I didn't want any bloodwork drawn because we weren't going to treat anything. Surprisingly, Dr. X agreed and said he would do the same thing. However, he was still talking about her nutrition. Mom weighs 101.5 pounds with all her clothes*

on. I told him that I don't care about her weight. If she is hungry, I want her to have food. If she doesn't want to eat, that is okay. Hopefully, it helps to keep verifying what the game plan is.

Harbinger of the End

One Sunday in March of 2013, we noticed that Mom had not swallowed a small bite of food she had taken at the restaurant and was still chewing it upon return to Oakwood. Peter noted the same phenomenon the following day. Subsequently, I sent the following email to my siblings.

> *I spoke to Peggy Brennan* [my husband's sister] *who is a speech therapist and specializes in swallowing. Peggy explained that there are more than fifty muscles involved in swallowing and four stages. The stages include seeing the fork and food on the table, deciding to pick up the fork, use it to gather food, move the food to your mouth, open your mouth, and put the food in it. We learn how to eat as babies, with this sequence being the first thing we learn and the last thing to go. Next, we chew the food and swallow. These are all voluntary actions. The rest of the process is involuntary, as*

the food moves down the esophagus and into the stomach. Peggy says that Mom doesn't have the attention span to remember the rest of the voluntary process. She literally forgets to swallow. In addition, since there are so many muscles involved, they are getting weaker and not working properly, so it is easier to aspirate and/or choke. Pneumonia is a common complication for this reason. Peggy thinks that Mom is further along in the dying process— "transitional" in her assessment via phone.

Peter, the more I think about it, I don't think it advisable to do the Big Boy on Sunday. It was SO hard last week and now we have incontinence in the picture as well. It is more than we can handle to take her out. It might be better now for you and me to stagger our visits too, so that I can check on her at other times and we have a family member there to keep an eye on her condition every few days.

As hard as it was taking her out on Sunday, I'm glad in hindsight that we did it. Had we decided that, because of her cough and the bitter cold, we should not take her out, I think we might have missed the whole picture of what is happening. I feel very reassured that Oakwood has stepped up their surveillance and level of care. I do feel she is being well cared for, kept clean, not going hungry or thirsty if she wants to eat or drink, and that our expressed wishes are being followed. She does not seem to be in any pain or distress.

I have since learned that 'pocketing' of food in the mouth or being unable to swallow is a late-stage symptom of dementia, signaling that death is not far off. It indicates that the body is beginning to shut down. Contrary to common belief, *sick people do not die because they stop eating; they stop eating because they are dying.* If food is forced on them at this time, their body cannot digest it, resulting in a variety of metabolic imbalances and often increasing discomfort and pain.

This fact goes contrary to every instinct we have as human beings. Food is life. Food is love. We feed those who cannot feed themselves. When a person becomes ill, they often lose their appetite and stop eating. A restoration of health is signaled by a returning appetite. Only then can we stop worrying. So, it is perfectly understandable that our impulse is to want to

see our sick loved one take in nourishment
again.

Winding Down

Everyone talks about the sheer number of doctors' visits that seem to be necessary as we age. It is amazing how much time this all can take. Well into her eighties, my mother was remarkably healthy and self-reliant. When we took her car away, she was still in her apartment in the Independent Living wing of Oakwood Commons. After that, Peter and I began driving and accompanying her to the various appointments—ophthalmologist, dentist, skin doctor, GYN doctor, foot doctor, chiropractor. Once she moved to Assisted Living, the facility offered the option of paying caretakers to transport her. We used this service a couple of times early on, when Peter and I were both engaged, and I was grateful for the break. But I don't recall that it worked for long as Mom soon became too uncooperative and refused to go without either Peter or me cajoling her.

Email from Patty on 2/20/13

> *I have been worrying a bit about upcoming doctors' appointments. On Sunday, Mom did not know me and asked several times who I was. We all went out to breakfast, and she was in a great*

mood, 'wound up' even, but she did not know me, and I need to be careful now to not be too affectionate or overstep with her until she warms up to me. In any case, I don't know if I'm going to be able to get her to go to doctors' appointments anymore, certainly not reliably.

Email from Patty on 2/28/13

I got a call this afternoon from Dr. X at Oakwood Common. Not our favorite guy, given that he gave Peter a hard time about signing off on Mom's Social Security check, gave us a hard time about calling in hospice, and apparently is a fan of keeping 96-year-old folks with severe dementia alive by all available means, for as long as possible and trying to shame families who don't agree with this approach. But he will be guided by our wishes and acknowledged as much. He was calling to ask why we were involving him in Mom's care if we don't want to treat her ... there is no point. He went on to express that he thought: (a) she was dehydrated and under nourished (he has said the nutrition piece repeatedly, nothing new); (b) she has a cough; (c) she might even have pneumonia; (d) her dementia is much worse, and he thought she should be moved to the Dementia Unit at Oakwood. (Apparently, Dr. X is unaware of the new philosophy regarding keeping people in place whenever possible.) His main point seemed to be that there was no point in him seeing her if we did not want her treated. I couldn't agree more (and Joan is on the same page).

Today Joan was unavailable for a short period of time during a series of calls back and forth as I tried to determine why Mom was taken to the clinic by the nurse in the first place. Turns out, there was a message on Joan's answering machine at home. Mom fell today. Unless she is in hospice, this will always trigger a medical response on Oakwood's part. Thankfully, they did not take her to the hospital. They also wanted Dr. X to see her and sign off on the fact that Mom is refusing all medications at this point, including her eyedrops (some internal policy that this must be documented).

Joan will follow up tomorrow with the nurse, with whom we still have not spoken. My intuition is that something is *going on with Mom. They found her on the floor earlier this week. Now another fall. For part of last Sunday, she did not know Peter. Maybe we'll call in another hospice evaluation. I'm guessing she would pass the can't-put-five-words-together dementia test at this point. The main advantage to having them involved is that Oakwood would not keep hauling her off to doctors and then we can just increase her level of care and frequency as needed. If she is a little sick right now (cough), it's not surprising that it might cause her to drink and eat less and get weaker, causing the falls, and so on. We have seen this spiral before. The thing that is different now, in my mind, is that she is losing her connection with her children, and I have long felt that we are what still anchors her here.*

Email from Peter on 3/4/13

Mother is now under hospice care.

Email from Patty on 5/15/13

Just thought I would share a few impressions with you. Physically, Mom is better than she was when we called in hospice in March, though in the last week, there have been two incidents: (1) bumped and scraped her arm and was taken to Oakwood for stitches (Peter and I were notified after the fact) and (2) Peter was called today about another relatively minor stumble and bruise. This sort of stuff seems to happen when she is weaker for some reason (dehydration, cough, not feeling well). I guess we can conclude that she is weaker overall and deteriorating physically, with an occasional rally here and there. Peter and I discussed this today. We had been thinking in the last couple of weeks it was possible she might be discharged from hospice again because so many of the former symptoms (swallowing difficulties, the cough, tendency to fall, lack of ambulation) had improved. We both agreed today that this seems unlikely now.

She is ambulatory. She has continence issues, but is not fully incontinent, according to the nurse. Aides are bathing and dressing her and doing all personal care now. Because they have taken this over, some of the issues have improved and she tends to look clean and appropriately dressed now (if you discount the size 18 skirt and sweater outfit that Peter and Chris found her dressed in on Mother's Day from God know where). We're hypothesizing that whatever closet these came out of perhaps houses the rest of Mom's missing clothes/sweaters, in which case, that lady's family is probably equally puzzled about how they are supposed to fit their size eighteen mother into size eight petite clothes.

My impression is that you all would find Mom shockingly worse mentally. I see a big decline here. She now spends a great deal of her time sitting at her table in the dining room. This is a switch from sitting in the hallway near the dining room which she had been doing for the past few months. Apparently, she was constantly challenging and defeating the ropes designed to keep folks out of the dining room until mealtime. Staff has conceded that she can sit there if she wants.

On Mother's Day, that is where I found her at 2:30 in the afternoon (keep in mind that lunch concludes at 12:30 and dinner starts at 4:30). She was examining the hem of the tablecloth the entire time I visited. She did not know me and only occasionally glanced up from her preoccupation. I brought flowers and sat with her for a short while. She could not understand why I was there. I can't explain the way she looks at me, but it is so strange and makes me feel sad. When I tried to bring her attention to the flowers (in the past, this helped her connect with the idea that it was me, or at least something familiar), she finally said "very pretty" because she seemed to get that I expected some kind of response. I decided to make my way down to her apartment to clean up (as Peter had reported it was a complete mess that morning) and put the flowers in a vase. I found the apartment in good shape, so staff must have come in and cleaned it up. I did not bother saying goodbye when I left. I was tempted to cry, but it takes too much out of me, and I stuffed it wherever I put this and went about the rest of my day. It's just very hard to go there and feel that I cannot bring her a spark of joy or even distraction. For a long time, we have been reporting a holding pattern, with a slow decline. That is not the case anymore.

Post-script: Indeed, it was no longer the case. Soon thereafter, Dorothy fell again, this time fracturing her hip. She took to her bed, under hospice care, and died a week later, on May 31, 2013.

Tips for Caregivers—Take-Away Lessons

- ✓ Remember that emotions become more important than logic.
- ✓ Understand that the person is acting in a way that this consistent with their reality. Be curious about that 'reality' and empathize with their experience.
- ✓ Try to evoke positive emotions or sensory experiences.
- ✓ Create and reinforce simple rituals and routines. Consistency will help to maintain a sense of familiarity.

As your loved one's symptoms progress, you will need to modify your behavior. For example, in response to vision changes, you might notice that a person with dementia startles easily. This may be at least in part due to a loss of peripheral vision. It may help to:

- ✓ Announce your presence.
- ✓ Narrate what you are doing.
- ✓ Stay in their line of sight.

Communicating with a Person Who Has Dementia	
Never	**Instead ...**
Correct	Let it pass
Argue	Agree
Reason	Divert; calm reassurance
Shame	Distract
Lecture	Reassure
Say "I told you"	Repeat; regroup
Say "you can't"	Focus on what they CAN
Command/demand	Ask/model
Condescend	Encourage
Force	Reinforce

Two Simple Ideas

➢ One family created a 'busy box' for their father. It contained various belongings that he liked to touch, hold, and fiddle with, providing hours of entertainment.

➢ Towards the end of his life, Ronald Reagan reportedly occupied himself by meticulously fishing leaves out of his swimming pool with a net. The attending Secret Service folks would round up the leaves and put them back in the pool when he wasn't looking, keeping him happily occupied.

Meeting the Emotional Challenges— What Helped Me

- ✓ Nonjudgment (for myself and others); accepting that feelings are feelings, neither right nor wrong; and that we all have our own way of coping
- ✓ Laughing, dark humor
- ✓ Phone calls with Joan
- ✓ Joining forces with siblings for some visits rather than always making a solo trip (while understanding this is not the best strategy for providing coverage overall, but still worth it to reduce the sense of burden and make visits more fun)
- ✓ Mourning the benchmarks and validating the losses as they happen; dementia involves a series of losses; often referred to as 'the long goodbye'
- ✓ Slowing down, finding some joy in the moment
- ✓ Instead of focusing on what we CAN'T do together, think "what CAN we do?" Take

her for a walk or a ride in the car? Watch
the birds, the flowers, the traffic? Go on a
'picnic?'

✓ Reconciling feelings of relief with grief—
they go hand in hand and that's okay; it's
normal and doesn't need to be fixed

That Was a Death

The day I realized there was no longer any point
in telling Mom about my life
Expecting her to hold the thread of my story
To keep up, to feel pride
Like expecting a three-year-old to meet your
needs
She cannot comprehend, and I best change
gears (again)
And think of how to amuse her
(Always easier when Peter was present)
That was a death.

Trying to make a connection
She's in her own world now.
I join her in her spot in the hallway
Pulling up a chair
Another resident witnesses her rebuffs, her lack
of recognition
And kindly says,
She doesn't know you.
I surprise myself, bursting into tears.
That was a death.

INTO THE FOG

A Mother's Day low, two weeks before she died
We have run the gamut from forgetful, to
confused, and beyond.
Puzzled, foggy, muddled, baffled, mystified,
perplexed, befuddled ...
Escalating to incomprehensible, lost
Until finally this: Vacant
Uncomprehending eyes, incapable of joy
I impose a kiss on her as I leave (after all, it is
Mother's Day!)
I know the kiss is more for me than for her.
That was a death.

She was always my friend
Always on my side
Now I am losing her, bit by bit,
My friend is gone.
In her place: Shadow Mom, as John would say
Relentless progression towards an inevitable
end
So many losses along the way
Once she is released from this broken shell
A flood of relief settles in.

I'm Not Gonna Miss You

*by Glen Campbell**

I'm still here, but yet I'm gone
I don't play guitar or sing my songs
They never defined who I am
The man that loves you 'til the end

You're the last person I will love
You're the last face I will recall
And best of all, I'm not gonna miss you
Not gonna miss you

I'm never gonna hold you like I did
Or say I love you to the kids
You're never gonna see it in my eyes
It's not gonna hurt me when you cry

I'm never gonna know what you go through
All the things I say or do
All the hurt and all the pain
One thing selfishly remains

I'm not gonna miss you
I'm not gonna miss you

*In his final music video, released three years prior to his death, Glenn performed this heartbreaking song. He died of Alzheimer's disease on August 8, 2017.

Dorothy's Death—A Cherished Memory

Mom had been readmitted to hospice care in mid-March that year. After my horrible Mother's Day visit, her decline accelerated. There were a couple of falls and an ER visit for stitches. And then she had a more serious fall and fractured her hip, signaling the beginning of the end. She went to bed, never to get up again.

In the last week, as Mom was dying, Joan shared that she feared the dying process, how it would unfold. Peter responded that he didn't care about that. He feared her death, losing her, finally. I don't remember feeling afraid. I just wanted the struggle to be over.

We all took turns at her bedside mixed with packing up her things. As a business owner, I could only afford to take limited time off from work. The prospect of packing things up for days *after* she died was prohibitive. Joan, having used up most of her paid time off with frequent visits over the past couple of years, also needed to return to Florida and to work promptly. John was off the grid, away on an expedition trekking across an ice flow in Alaska. This long-planned trip involved a group of people and a considerable investment of time and money. Receiving word of her now imminent death a day or two prior to leaving for the trip, John made the decision to proceed to Alaska. He would join us afterwards if it wasn't too late. So it was that John was not with us when Mom died. But a remarkable thing happened to offset his absence.

Dorothy, at first responsive to us, began to slip further and further away as the week progressed, until she was a mostly inert presence on the bed. It was all very peaceful, but her breathing became labored. My son Terry was Dorothy's firstborn grandchild and the only grandchild for the first four years of his life, thereby securing a special place in her heart. He called me every day that week, asking for updates. He seemed especially tuned in to what was unfolding a 45-minute drive away. He repeatedly asked whether I "needed" him to come. Regretfully, I remember responding that I didn't feel *I needed* him to come but if he wanted to, he was certainly welcome. And then the next day, we would have the same conversation, and he would ask the same question. By the third round, I finally came up with a different answer, reflecting that it seemed to me that *he wanted* to be present with us and, if that was the case, he had best do it today or tomorrow because her death was close.

The next day, late in the afternoon, Terry arrived. Chris was there too, and we were all together. Dorothy's breathing had become even more labored. As it was late in the afternoon, we were all done packing for the day, and everyone was getting hungry. Peter and Terry left to pick up Chinese takeout for dinner. Meanwhile, the rest of us arranged ourselves in a circle around Mom's bed. Joan and I were positioned on either side of her, near the head of the bed, each of us holding a hand. And Mike and Chris had taken up their seats around the bed. I can't remember another time throughout the week when all of us were so together, so present, and so focused on her. Peter and Terry returned with the food and came to stand in the bedroom doorway, near the foot of the bed. Then, at that moment, a most unexpected thing occurred. Roberta, my brother John's wife, called to check in. We put Roberta on speaker and laid the phone on Mom's belly, as it was the most central spot in the room. And then Dorothy breathed her last breath. So, Roberta was 'there,' both present with us and as a proxy for John. The maximum number of loved ones who could be present, were indeed fully present at the moment of death. I experienced this as an extraordinary blessing. Did Mom choose her moment of death? (It certainly seems so.) If so, how does that work? As Terry came to sit next to me on my stool and put his arm around me, I briefly felt a shudder of electric impulses through my hand, still holding Mom's hand, which confused me momentarily. A final discharge of energy from the body. And in that moment, I was overcome with gratitude for Terry's presence and this remarkable ending. It turns out I did need him there, and I believe she waited for him as well. When asked, days later, for his impression of the experience, Terry summed up his feelings in one word—"profound."

Epilogue: Perspective Returns

In the years when my mother was first failing, and then mostly gone, I remember wondering whether I would ever get to a point when I could think of her and remember better days and not just the process of losing her, little by little, over six years. The weight of it was crushing at times. Would the vacant eyes haunt me, holding fast in my mind, and forever dominate my memories of her? Would this be her true legacy? I worried about this (needlessly, as is true of most worrying).

It took a couple of years or so for perspective to return. In the beginning, shortly after her death, the whole ordeal dominated my thoughts and memories of her. Eventually, however, I can now testify that memories of happier times, times of connection and friendship have returned. In fact, the good memories dominate. The story of her decline is decidedly not the whole story. Not for her, not for any of us. It just feels that way sometimes.

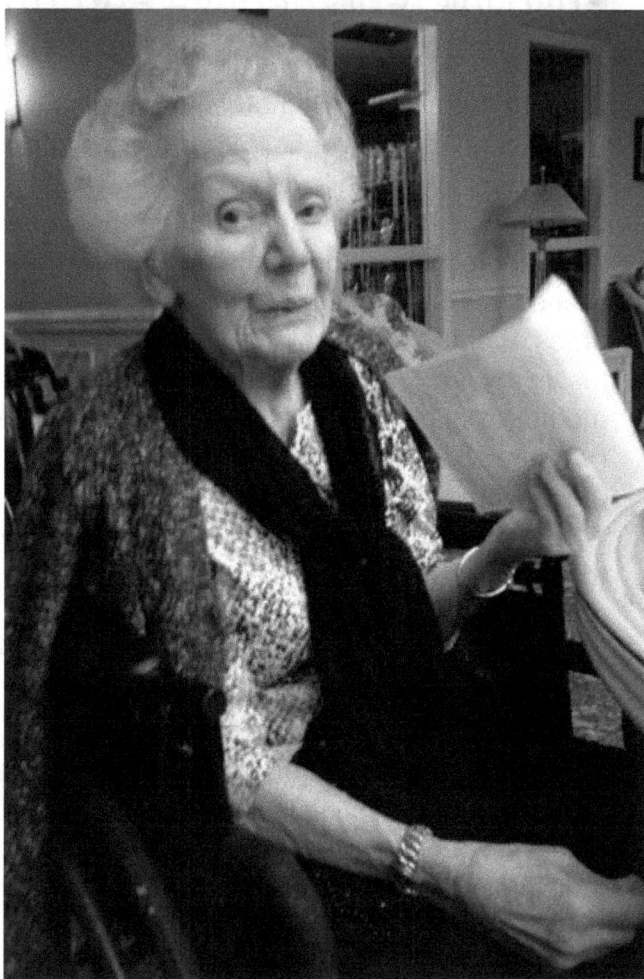

Dorothy Marie Sweeney McInerney
December 16, 1916–May 31, 2013

Appendix A
A Brief Primer on Dementia

Dementia is the loss of cognitive functioning to such an extent that it interferes with a person's daily life and activities. It is characterized by impairment of at least two brain functions, such as memory loss and judgment. Symptoms include forgetfulness, limited social skills, loss of speech, impaired problem-solving ability, and more. While there are some treatments available to help manage the symptoms of dementia, there is no cure. It is a progressive disease.

There are several types of dementia: Alzheimer's disease, vascular dementia, Lewy body dementia, frontotemporal dementia, mixed dementia (with one or more causes), and other rarer types. While Alzheimer's is the most frequently diagnosed form of dementia, the terms *dementia* and *Alzheimer's* are often used interchangeably, though this is not accurate. There is abundant information online regarding the distinct types of dementia and associated symptoms, summarized by folks with lots more experience in the field than I have. I don't see the point of repeating such readily available information here but encourage you to dive in online if your loved one has a specific diagnosis and you seek a more detailed understanding of their disease trajectory. From the individual's and family's perspective navigating this disease, I don't know that the labels matter so much.

Some common symptoms of dementia include:

- Loss of reason and logic, confusion, delusions; emotions become dominant and stronger
- Loss of memory, especially short-term memory
- Difficulty communicating with loss of vocabulary and speech comprehension; person uses the wrong word, loses their train of thought, or becomes frustrated searching for words
- Changes in vision include loss of peripheral vision, aka 'tunnel vision' or 'scuba view' (must be directly in front of them); may lose ability to detect form (e.g., faces), color, motion, light, shadow, reflection; caregivers may notice that the person startles easily
- Sleep disturbances, motor impairment, and incontinence may be involved.

Stages of Dementia

The symptoms of dementia will keep changing so caregivers will need to adapt their support efforts as the disease progresses. As a general guide, we can group the progression of symptoms as follows:

Mild Dementia. The person may frequently lose the ability to remember what just happened to them. Routine tasks become difficult, such as cooking. Some tasks can become more dangerous, such as driving.

Moderate Dementia. Communication becomes extremely limited. The person loses the ability to understand what is going on around them and requires daily assistance with dressing and often toileting. Some people can become quite confused, agitated, and paranoid while others are content much of the time.

Advanced Dementia. Sufferers are no longer able to recognize loved ones and family members. Some people with severe dementia may be calm and serene much of the time, but many go through periods of agitation. They can be awake through the night. They can be angry, disruptive, and yelling. Eventually, they need 24-hour help with all daily activities, including

bathing and assistance with all basic body
functions.

Appendix B

Understanding Hospice Care

Because most folks enter hospice care within a week or two of their death, there is widespread misunderstanding about hospice. In fact, hospice care is designed to support anyone with a diagnosis of an incurable disease who is not receiving life-extending treatments and is expected to die within six months if the disease takes its normal course. While there are a few live-in hospice facilities for folks who are in the active phase of dying, most hospice care today is provided by the family at home, under the guidance of the hospice team. It is a shame that people are so hesitant to enter hospice care. Family caregivers might afford themselves a break, getting some much-needed help from the hospice team. For example, hospice care includes three weekly visits from a home health aide to assist with showering. It has been shown that people live longer when under hospice care.

Curative Care versus Hospice Care

Curative Care	Hospice Care
Goal is to treat the disease and extend life; emphasis on quantity, not quality.	Goal is to treat the whole person; help people have the fullest possible life now; emphasis on quality, not quantity.
Treats the patient only.	Patient and family form the unit of care.
May sacrifice quality of life now (through chemotherapy, surgery, etc.) for the chance of gaining time later.	Focus on freedom from pain and discomfort, maintaining mental awareness, spending time with family, etc.

What is Hospice?

- A form of palliative care specific to end of life
- Care focused on comfort and improving quality of life

- A multidisciplinary care team approach that includes a doctor, nurse case manager, social worker, chaplain, home health aides (up to three visits per week), volunteers, and bereavement support
- Expert management of symptoms; keep the dying comfortable, manage pain
- May receive care wherever they live Skilled Nursing Care facility); few in-patient hospice facilities exist; most care is in the home and family provides 24-hour care
- 24-hour on-call service for telephone or in-home support by a nurse
- Addresses physical, emotional, mental, and spiritual aspects of living with a terminal diagnosis
- Helps patient and family prepare for a peaceful death; keeps the death from becoming an emergency event (no need to call 911 when person dies)

Additional Services Provided

- Short-term respite care (up to five days)
- Short-term in-patient services (for pain and symptom management)
- Prescription medications

- Medical equipment (e.g., bed, commode, wheelchair, walker, etc.)
- Medical supplies (e.g., bandages, catheters, etc.)
- Grief/bereavement counseling and support for adults and children up to 13 months after the death; open to all, even if family did not use hospice services prior to the death

Qualifications for Hospice

- Anyone, regardless of ability to pay is eligible; hospice is a covered benefit under Medicaid/ Medicare and all private insurance companies.
- Two physicians have verified that if the disease follows the expected course, the patient has six months or less to live.
- Patient is choosing to forego curative treatments like surgery or chemo, unless these are deemed necessary for comfort.
- For anyone who wants a peaceful death and has chosen to not pursue further medical treatments aimed at extending life
- An individual/family can choose to discontinue hospice care at any time; may also return to hospice when eligible.

- Patient must be recertified as hospice eligible every six months; may be discharged from hospice if health improves.

Hospice Eligibility Criteria for Dementia Patients

Since dementia doesn't play by the same rules as other diseases at the end of life, it is harder to predict when the dementia patient will become eligible for hospice care. The Functional Assessment Staging Test or FAST scale is a crucial tool in hospice care for quantifying the progression of dementia. It measures the decline in dementia patients, providing a standardized way to document changes over time. Once the patient is at or beyond stage 7 of the FAST scale, they are hospice eligible and may meet any or all the following criteria:

- The patient is unable to move independently and requires assistance.
- The patient is unable to bathe or dress themselves without assistance.
- The patient has bowel and/or bladder incontinence.
- The patient is unable to speak or communicate meaningfully. This may

include being limited to six or fewer intelligible words a day.

- The patient has had one of the following within the past 12 months: aspiration pneumonia, pyelonephritis or other upper urinary tract infection, septicemia, or multiple stage 3–4 decubitus ulcers.
- The patient has lost 10 percent of their weight in the previous six months.
- The patient has a serum albumin of less than 2.5 gm/dl. (Serum albumin is a protein found in blood plasma).

Appendix C

Introduction to Advance Care Planning (ACP)

Standard of Care

The current standard of care during a medical emergency (when the patient cannot communicate) is to do everything possible to save someone's life unless *there is a medical order to the contrary*. Lifesaving interventions may include CPR, intubation, dialysis, tube feeding, intensive care, and so on. If an individual does not want the standard of care applied, then advance care planning will help ensure the person's preferences are honored.

What is ACP?

ACP is a process of communication and documentation that helps individuals at any stage of health or illness to:

1. Identify a healthcare advocate and alternate advocate whom they appoint to make medical decisions on their behalf should they become unable to do so (Medical Power of Attorney, aka Health Care Proxy), and
2. Discuss their values and wishes for the

end of life with their advocates and loved ones (aka Living Will).

To be effective, this process of communication needs to be individualized, based on a person's state of health, and updated whenever health status changes or other conditions such as a death, divorce, or relocation occur (or at least every five years).

In the United States, laws governing the ACP process vary from state to state. The required legal documents may go by different names such as Advance Directive (AD) or Health Care Power of Attorney, depending on the state you live in. In some instances, medical orders can be part of the ACP documentation. POLST forms (portable medical orders) and Do Not Resuscitate (DNR) orders are created and signed by health care providers and give specific medical treatment orders to other providers based on the individual's wishes. *These are only issued when the patient is extremely sick or frail, in the late stages of a disease.*

The only legally binding component of an AD is the designation of the medical advocate or proxy. Few people realize that the individual's expressed wishes are designed to provide guidance to their advocate but are not legally binding. Hence the need for Medical Orders to be added to the documentation as the person's illness progresses. Many families (including mine) have been unpleasantly surprised when an AD was ignored in a crisis because the medical proxy was not on hand to advocate.

The single most important thing people can do to ensure their wishes are honored is to have a conversation about their preferences with all key family members. Your medical advocate needs to have a thorough understanding of what you want and WHY. If all other family members can support the advocate in their decision making, then there is the possibility of peaceful acceptance, even if everyone is not on the same page about the choices being made. If not, then there will likely be hard feelings, guilt, and worse among loved ones.

Finally, the ACP process includes dissemination of the documents to appropriate parties, such as your physician, hospital or health system, advocate(s), neighbors or other close friends, and anyone who might be involved or notified when a health crisis occurs. It is recommended that copies of the documents be kept in readily accessible locations such as a file drawer, glove box or suitcase when traveling, and that a wallet card direct emergency personnel to these locations.

What are we trying to accomplish and why?

When someone has been diagnosed with a life-limiting illness, a Living Will can be created by engaging in a conversation around the following questions regarding their values and wishes:

- What is your understanding of your condition or prognosis?
- What are your fears or worries about what lies ahead?
- What goals do you have as your time gets short? How do you want to spend your time?
- What are you willing to trade off or sacrifice, for the sake of having more time? How much suffering are you willing to go through?
- What outcomes are unacceptable to you?
- How do you define "quality of life"? What would a good day look like?

When caregivers are pushing eating and sleeping, and forcing activities for a person who is at the end of life, the key question is: *What are we trying to accomplish and why?* What is the outcome for which we are hoping? Notice whether, when forcing someone to eat and get out of bed, they are complying gently or are unhappy and discontent. If they are displaying unhappiness and discontent, why would we want to make their days miserable?

Challenges to Honoring Advanced Directives

Be aware that if the person is living in a nursing home or Assisted Living facility, institutional policies and protocols may trump an AD. For example, at one stage, my mom was in an Assisted Living facility with moderate-to-advanced dementia but was not eligible for hospice care. The facility had a non-negotiable protocol to transport to the ER any resident who experienced a fall. The family, following my mother's wishes, had no intention of treating any injuries from a fall (short of stitching her up if she were bleeding), but we could not circumvent this requirement until Mom was determined to be hospice eligible. Hence, my brother made numerous (unnecessary, in our view) trips to the ER.

In addition, institutional routines can often override the expressed wishes of the individual and family as the default mode of operation. For example, caregivers in a nursing home—whose job it is to get the patients in their care fed, dressed, and out of bed—may find it difficult to honor requests to refrain from cajoling/coercing patients into eating at the end of life. Family advocacy may be required to ensure that the patient's wishes are honored.

How is an Ethical Will different from a Living Will?

An Ethical Will is a written document in a narrative and highly individual format that expresses a person s goals, values, and wishes concerning how they live and how they want to die. It can also include moral imperatives and statements of concern, forgiveness, or permission, as well as blessings and wisdom one wants to pass on to the next generation. Creating an ethical will can be a very meaningful process, like life review or a legacy project.

An ethical will should not be confused with a living will. A living will form is often included in the various AD packages and focuses specifically on healthcare choices at the end of life. Some living will forms may simply contain lists of options accompanied by a check box. An ethical will, on the other hand, may be conceived of as a letter, audio recording, or video. It serves as a legacy gift for the family.

Advance Directives for Dementia Patients

In the Resources following I share several online tools that will walk you through your choices and preferences for care if you or someone you love has dementia. The tools can be used to generate specific guidance to loved ones regarding your wishes. A common theme is that people say they no longer wish to live if they can't recognize family members but it's important to unpack that statement. Does 'recognize' mean they remember names and relationships? What about recognizing a familiar face that loves you and makes you feel special, even if you can't place the person? It all comes down to each person's definition of quality of life.

Summary

Advanced Directive
- ✓ Includes a Durable Medical Power of Attorney (POA)* designate
- ✓ Can be completed anytime
- ✓ Requires no medical signatures
- ✓ Not legally binding (only POA is binding)
- ✓ Only applicable when we cannot speak for ourselves

* There are two kinds of Durable Power of Attorney—one for finances and one for medical decisions

Physician Orders for Life Sustaining Treatment (POLST)
- ✓ Each state has its own version and may go by other names.
- ✓ Guides first responders and physicians regarding types of life-sustaining treatments you want
- ✓ It is a legal medical order.
- ✓ Must be completed and signed by health care provider
- ✓ Created for the seriously ill, frail, elderly

No Code 911
- ✓ aka Allow Natural Death (AND)
- ✓ aka Do Not Resuscitate (DNR)
- ✓ aka Do Not Attempt Resuscitation (DNAR)
- ✓ aka No Code
- ✓ Legal order signed by a physician
- ✓ Typically, order is given when the person is so gravely ill that death is imminent and inevitable.

Resources

Gawandi, Atul. *Being Mortal.* (2017). I highly recommend this book as you consider the issue of quantity versus quality of life, from the perspective of a physician.

Karnes, Barbara. *How Do I Know You? Dementia at the End-of-Life* and *Always Offer, Never Force: Food at the End of Life.* Educational booklets focused on the challenges present in the weeks to days before a person with dementia dies. These materials bring perspective to considerations regarding tube feeding, forced hand feeding, and artificial hydration at the end of life. Available from https://bkbooks.com/collections. Barbara Karnes is a well-known hospice nurse, pioneer of the hospice movement, end-of-life educator, and author. She is the author of "the little blue book" *(Gone from My Sight)* that all hospices provide to families in their care as an educational tool to understand the dying process.

Helpful Web-Based Resources

Alzheimer's Association
https://www.alz.org/
Free in-person and virtual support groups for family caregivers, limited financial support (who knew?!), information, and advocacy.

American Association of Retired Persons (AARP)
https://www.aarp.org/caregiving/
Resources for family caregivers.

Michigan's Guide for Aging Drivers and their Families.
https://www.michigan.gov/agingdriver
https://www.alz.org/help-support/caregiving/safety/dementia-driving
The guide is a great resource for family caregivers. It emphasizes how aging affects the ability to drive safely. A portion of the guide includes information to help establish whether a person is safe to drive. Tools include a driving self-assessment, guidance on partnering with the medical community, and how to request a driver evaluation.

Advance Directives

Caring Info
https://www.caringinfo.org/planning/advance-directives/by-state/
Download your state's advance directives.

Compassion and Choices
https://compassionandchoices.org/dementia-values-tool/
Offers a Dementia Values and Priorities Tool.

Conversation Project
https://theconversationproject.org/
Offers several free guides, from a "Conversation Starter Guide" to "Choosing a Health Care Proxy," and more. They also have a "Conversation Starter Guide for Caregivers of People with Alzheimer's or Other Forms of Dementia."

Dementia Directive
https://dementia-directive.org/
Here is another form summarizing considerations for documenting your wishes as the disease progresses.

Final Exit Network
https://finalexitnetwork.org/

- Offers a Dementia Provision (Advance Directive Addendum) that includes guidance designed to prevent dying people from being hand fed against their wishes.
- Also offers an "Advance Directive for Voluntary Stopping of Eating and Drinking (VSED)" which is only an option for folks in the early stages of dementia.

Five Wishes
https://www.fivewishes.org/for-myself/
Digital tools customized to meet requirements in all fifty states. Allows you to make unlimited revisions without any time limits. Also available in print form.

POLST (Physician's Orders for Life-Sustaining Treatment)
https://polst.org/programs-in-your-state/
Look for a POLST program in your state (sometimes goes by other names than POLST).

About the Author

Patty Brennan was born in 1952 in Detroit, Michigan. She is the fourth child of five born to Bernie and Dorothy McInerney over a seven-year period—Mike, Peter, Joan, Patty, and John. Patty grew up in Dearborn, Michigan and went to St. Mary's College in South Bend, Indiana and Boston College, graduating in 1974 with a liberal arts degree. In 1977, she moved to Ann Arbor, Michigan where she lives today. Patty married a childhood friend, Jerry Brennan in 1978 and they soon added sons Terry and Max and, eventually, six grandchildren to their family.

Patty has been self-employed her entire adult life. Following an unconventional path to become a direct-entry homebirth midwife, she also trained as a childbirth educator and doula and worked to support families in a process of informed decision-making and proactive planning for the upcoming birth of their baby. Her work continuously evolved over the years, eventually retiring from being 'on-call' for births to become a doula trainer and founder of a community-based nonprofit organization featuring a volunteer doula program known as *Doulas Care*. An estimated 250 low-income families per year were served by the program under Patty's leadership over a nine-year period.

In 2010, Patty published *The Doula Business Guide* to provide step-by-step guidance for new doulas to establish viable businesses. The book was followed by *The Doula Business Guide Workbook* in 2016. These books have been updated every few years since, with the latest fourth edition published in early 2024.

After losing two sets of parents and witnessing the remarkable similarities between the processes of birthing and dying, Patty added end-of-life doula training to her curricula, launching the first end-of-life doula training in Michigan in 2016. She founded Lifespan Doulas [www.LifespanDoulas.com] in 2019 and continues to be fully engaged in the business today, offering online birth, postpartum, and end-of-life doula training, certification, and business development guidance for doulas. She is available as a speaker on end-of-life topics and the doula model of care, and serves as a trainer/consultant for hospices, palliative care clinical teams, and home health agencies seeking to get staff trained as doulas or to establish doula programs. Patty may be contacted via email, *patty@lifespandoulas.com*.